TAMING THE
STORY OF A \

Richard Horuk

Chapter 1 Introduction

Wegener's Granulomatosis is an autoimmune disease that is caused by inflammation of the small blood vessels. It can be a devastating and lethal disease depending on which of the body's tissues and organs it affects. Like most autoimmune diseases Wegener's is probably induced in multiple ways, including infectious agents, genetic predisposition, environmental factors, etc. The exact triggers of the disease still remain unknown but there has been much speculation into the root causes. Whatever the exact mechanisms of the disease, the treatments can be equally as brutal as the disease itself. These include giving the patient infusions of cellular poisons like cyclophosphamide (Cytoxan is a chemotherapeutic agent often used in the treatment of cancer patients) together with massive doses of steroids. The first few chapters of this book will be devoted to discussing the disease, it's treatments, and it's clinical outcomes in more depth. But first I would like to start with my own personal history to illustrate how one seemingly innocuous moment changed my life forever.

My name is Richard Horuk, and my story revolves around my battles with Wegener's. I was born in 1947 in a small village called Salzgitter- Lebenstedt, in what was then, West Germany. My mother was German and together with my grandmother, had fled her home in East Prussia ahead of the advancing Soviet army during the end of the Second World War. They endured some rough times while traversing the war ravaged German countryside ending up in Lebenstedt, which became part of the British occupation zone. It was in this small village that my mother met my father. My dad was Ukrainian and he had fought with the Germans against their common Russian enemies. When the war ended, my father had no country because the Ukraine was absorbed into the Soviet empire. Consequently, my dad lived in Lebenstedt in a camp together with all of the other homeless and stateless citizens of Europe, whose numbers had grown increasingly as a consequence of the war. My father tried to find work in Germany after the war ended but because he was a foreign national, and a stateless one at that, it proved to be impossible. He had no passport and no prospects other than to participate in Black Market activities just to feed himself. Europe in those early post-war days was a most inhospitable place to live and to move in freely. What a stark contrast to the ease of travel that we all take for granted today!

Thus it was that I lived in Lebenstedt for almost 4 years, with my mother and grandmother because my father had decided that he needed to leave Germany to secure a job and steady income. The choices at that time were basically England or Canada. Although my dad had relatives in Canada, my mother refused to consider to go there because it was too far away from her only remaining parent, my Grandmother, who lived in Germany. My Grandfather had gone missing in the war on the Eastern Front and was never seen or heard of again, one of the many millions that the war had taken. One of my earliest recollections of those first few years living without my dad was the memory of receiving packages from him filled with food and clothes. My mom told me they were from my dad and I used to think that the postman who delivered them to our house was my dad!

My father told me that when he landed in England, it was equally challenging to find work and he lived in several camps around the country together with other stateless persons. As jobs were scarce in those early post-war years, the choice as he tells it was either to work as a field hand for a farmer or to go down into the coal mines. No real job opportunities or training programs in those dreary days. The choice for him was simple; mining paid well and farming did not. Thus it was that he found temporary jobs as a coal miner in various mines throughout the UK until he finally got a permanent position as a *"face"* worker in a mine in Derbyshire called Cossall Colliery. Cossall was a drift mine, which meant you could walk down a very steep, incline to get to the pit face, no cage was required. However at the end of a long hard day working on the face hewing out coal and breathing in the filth and dust that the coal cutting machines produced, you had to walk up this incline to get out to the light of the outside world. As my father put it "if the hard days work didn't do you in, the walk out of the pit up the steep slope did". Once he was established in this position, in 1951, he decided the time was right to bring his family over. He made the long trek back to Germany to fetch his family and bring them back to his new homeland.

After a long tearful farewell with my grandmother and all my other relatives at a small railway station near our village, the three of us set off on our journey to England to a city called Nottingham. Nottingham is an industrial city that was the home of John Player, a company who manufactured cigarettes, Raleigh industries, who made bicycles, and the headquarters of Boots the chemists who are found in every town and city in the UK. In addition, the city is well known for producing exceedingly fine lace, however, it is more famous for the Sherriff of Nottingham and Robin Hood and is in an area of England called the Midlands. It was quite a contrast to the small village in Germany that I had just left.

It was strange to suddenly live in a country where I could not understand the language or the culture. Here I was living in the country of our victors wearing German clothes, i.e. "Lederhosen", and I got some strange and often hostile looks. Not unexpected, I guess, as the war against the Germans had only just ended six years ago. However, four-year olds adapt pretty quickly and within six months I was fluent not only in English but also in Ukrainian since we lived in an apartment in a house with other Ukrainian families. Within six months we moved into a home of our own, thanks to my Father working almost every hour that he could down in the mines. My parents managed to pay the mortgage and buy food and clothes, thanks to my dad's incredible work ethic and the fact that my Mother took in boarders cooking and cleaning for them to make ends meet. My parents worked really hard to make a decent life for their family and imbued me at an early stage with a strong work ethic and excellent values that have stayed with me all of my life and for which I cannot thank them enough.

I quickly adapted to life in England and at five-years old I started in the English school system. I progressed from the infant's school, five to seven-year olds, to the primary school, seven to eleven-year olds. I quickly mastered English literature and was extremely well read at an early stage thanks to the schoolteacher who lived next door to us. She supplied me with an endless treasure trove of the classics - Chaucer, Milton, Homer, Roman Myths and Legends, etc. Another neighbor who was an accountant helped me master mathematics so I had the basics covered at a very early age. My major problem at school was that I was easily bored, especially since I had already mastered most of the subjects that we were being taught. My reaction in this situation was simply to switch off and not participate in class. The teachers interpreted this as a sign of laziness and I was usually in trouble with one or more of them, and in their eyes I was not academically gifted. This label stuck with me throughout the rest of my time at primary school and quite likely influenced the entire course of my future education.

In those days, the British system had a final exam in primary school, called the "eleven plus". As its name suggests, this exam was taken at the age of eleven and it determined whether you went to a Grammar school, which was a pathway to University, if you passed, or to a secondary school and some menial or blue collar jobs if you failed the exam. The format of the exam was similar to IQ tests i.e. distinguish between these different shapes, or which one of these pictures is different, etc. It did not test my knowledge of Shakespeare or my mastery of Chaucer and the classics. Consequently, I perceived the exam as irrelevant and just switched off. I failed it with quite some style!

My next four years were thus spent at a secondary school, Huntingdon secondary modern, which had a reputation for being a school with a lot of tough kids who belonged to one local gang or another. Since some of these kids lived near us and I was friendly with them, I had an easier time at school than many of the other kids who were regularly harassed by these young hooligans. The secondary school was split into "academic streams" A, being the highest followed by B, C, and D. In each of the four years I progressed in the A stream going from 1A to 4A quite smoothly always managing to be in the middle of the class academically at exam time. I coasted through school this way without too much exertion. The teachers would put comments like "must try harder", or "obviously bright, must apply himself" on my school reports. I ignored all of these remarks since school did not challenge me and as far as I was concerned it was easier just to switch off and do the minimum and still end up 18th out of 36 in the exams. Ironically, I found science (Chemistry, Physics and Biology) the most unbearably boring of my academic studies, because the teachers who taught them were totally uninspiring and their lectures were, in my eyes, tedious at best.

Thus, I regularly switched off during science lessons, ignoring most of what was being taught and consistently failed those classes. I look back on this with some amusement since I ended up as a well respected scientist with a Ph.D.! But more of this later.

Although I hated school with a vengeance I made sure I had a good time outside of school. I belonged to a gang of kids who, other than when we were up to no good, had fun in winter tobogganing down the steep hill that we lived on missing lamp posts and careening in front of cars, missing being crushed under lorries by inches! On bonfire day (a British tradition held on each November the 5th to celebrate Guy Fawkes trying to blow up Parliament and the King!) we piled up rubbish in the streets and set fire to it on a huge bonfire with fireworks galore, I still bear the scars of a fireworks accident on my foot when I was eleven-years old. In summer I learned to swim by jumping into the deep end, almost nine foot of water, at the various outdoor swimming pools in Nottingham. My friends and I indulged in a variety of lawless activities typical of unsupervised children in those days. If my parents had known half of what I got up to I am sure it would have turned their hair white.

My first taste of freedom came at the age of 15, when I left school against the wishes of my parents. My parents really wanted me to stay on in the fifth form and get better grades so I could pass the exams required for ultimately getting into University. At that time, the entry requirement for University in Britain was to obtain a General Certificate of Education or GCE. You needed five passes at the ordinary level, O-level, together with at least two passes at the advanced level, A-levels. However, at the age of 15 I was finished with the boredom of school and stubbornly refused to consider any more academic effort, regardless of how much my parents pushed me. To me the idea of wasting any more of my time enduring mind-numbing lessons was unfathomable. I wanted to go to work, earn money, and generally have a good time.

And so, my adulthood began. I spent the next six years working in a bookstore, this was a perfect job for me because I loved literature and interacting with people. During this time, I travelled throughout Europe, played a lot of snooker (a game similar to pool), indulged in all night card games and was generally having a good time. That said, my career was going nowhere. It was about this time at the age of 21 that I found out that some friends and acquaintances were getting college degrees. One was even pursing an advanced degree, a Ph. D. Suddenly I realized that although I was smarter than they were, they were going places and I was not. This was just the sort of 'kick in the pants' that I needed to get me re-motivated to pursue my education.

While I contemplated what discipline I would want to focus on when I returned to school, I decided a good challenge for me would be to change careers, moving away from literature. To really challenge myself, I decided to embark on a career in science. This might at first glance seem to be a strange choice since science was my weakest subject at school, however, I like to be challenged and this seemed like an appropriate goal to pursue. Besides which, I had become more interested in science from watching science programs on TV.

However my real interest in science especially chemistry was almost accidental, and came about as I was browsing through the bookshelves of our local library (no internet in those days people actually went to the library to slake their thirst for knowledge by borrowing books). One of the books that I pulled out at random was entitled "a compendium of useful formularies" or something like that. It had recipes for making cosmetics, soaps, paints, shoe polish, candles, etc. The book intrigued me and especially the many hundreds of recipes that gave detailed instructions on how to manufacture a variety of things like nail varnish, lip sticks, soap, shampoo, candles, shoe polish, etc, etc. I decided that I could follow the recipes and make some nail varnish and nail varnish remover and my friends and I could try to sell them to the small corner drug store at the top of the road. But how to get the chemicals to do this. Well I was pretty ingenious we had a garden shed in our backyard and I christened it the Acme Chemical Company and proceeded to buy chemicals from a local chemical supplier company in Nottingham. I even had chemicals delivered to our house by the suppliers so imagine my parents surprise when a van pulled up to our front door with supplies for the Acme Chemical Company. I reassured my parents that I was just pursuing an interest in science that might lead to a career and I think that they were so happy to see that I was actually thinking of pursuing something academic that they swallowed it hook line and sinker. I cannot imagine being able to do what I did then in the present era, too many safeguards thank goodness.

Thus it was that armed with countless bottles of chemicals too numerous to recount, but which included sulfuric, hydrochloric and nitric acids as well as some other highly dangerous and volatile compounds, I indulged my interest in chemistry. I made some nail varnish in various colors and was quite disappointed when the local drug store told me they were not interested in my wares. However, no problem since I had all of these chemicals now I used them to make explosives and various other interesting compounds. I guess I am lucky I didn't blow myself and my parents up during my many experiments in the garden shed. The net effect of all of this was that I was hooked on science it was like a drug I had to get more. I decided I could do this by trying to get a job in some sort of scientific position. This was not easy since I had no qualifications but I was determined to achieve my goal.

Thus it was that I managed to get a position in a dairy laboratory as a technician testing milk and dairy products for chemical composition and microbial contamination. I really enjoyed it and started doing little side projects in my spare time in the laboratory. I spent the next two years voraciously devouring every textbook on chemistry, microbiology and mathematics I could get my hands on, absorbing everything I read. At this time I took 5 GCE O-levels and passed them without ever going to formal classes, but purely by studying on my own! Things were humming along quite nicely. However, my plans were slightly disrupted at this time because my best friend and I were hanging around playing guitars and really enjoyed the experience. At about the same time I had left the dairy and got a job in a factory that produced Raleigh bikes, it was here that I met my first wife who had an absolutely beautiful voice, and the three of us formed a folk group playing songs by Bob Dylan and Joan Baez. We practiced hard and entered a talent contest unfortunately we did not win and decided that we would just play for fun.

My life changed again the following year when my daughter was born because now I had the responsibility of a wife and child to look after. Thus it was that I got a job in a soap factory as a technician testing soaps and cosmetics working eight hour shifts, either 6am to 2pm which I liked or 2pm to 10 pm which I hated or 10pm to 6am which allowed me to study during my work. I studied hard to get an A level in chemistry and passed the exam at the first attempt again without going to formal classes. However I would need an A level in another subject in order to have enough academic credit to enroll for a B. Sc. Degree. I decided why wait another two years to accomplish this and chose instead to enroll for what was then called a Higher National Diploma (HND). This was a two-year course and would, if I passed the exams, secure entry after completion into the B.Sc. degree. As it was, I was top of the entire class in the HND and after one year of study, they transferred me to year two of the B.Sc. class, majoring in biochemistry and microbiology. Three years later at the age of 27 I finally graduated with my Bachelors degree in science and I was absolutely delighted with what I had accomplished.

Armed with a B.Sc. degree I considered what I should do next. I had several options: get a job as a scientist (lab technician), do research for a higher degree, or go into medicine. After much thought, I decided to go into research as this was what really excited me, and I started applying for Ph.D. studentships at several universities. I was lucky enough to be accepted for a Ph.D. at three institutions: Warwick University, Glasgow University and the University of London. At Warwick my research project would be the study of microbial degradation of complex phenols, an important topic with potential applications in helping to clean up environmental pollutants. At Glasgow my research topic would be in the field of cancer research and at London the study of the molecular properties of insulin from a crystallographic approach. Given my background and interests the first two choices would have been the optimal ones, however, I chose London because it had a good rail connection to Nottingham. Since I had a wife and daughter, I decided that day to day commuting from Nottingham to London, a 2 hour journey by rail, would have the least impact on the family and would allow us to stay in Nottingham near our families. Thus it was that I embarked on a 3-year

CASE studentship at Birkbeck College at the University of London (under the mentorship of Professor Sir Thomas Blundell).

The most interesting aspect of this program was that it involved carrying out research at both the University of London and Burroughs Welcome, a pharmaceutical company in Dartford Kent (also a short rail journey south of London). This was fine with me because it would give me a taste of what it was like to be a scientist in industry. Despite the arduous daily commute and long hours, the next three years passed by very quickly. My research into insulin action and structure went well, culminating in receiving my Ph.D. in November 1980.

On reflection, it had been an interesting journey from being last in class at science in secondary school to getting a Ph.D. in science at the age of 32! My advisor, Tom, and I had long conversations about what I should do next and he gave me great advice, "go West young man" is in essence what he told me. With his help, I applied for and was successful in getting several Post-Doctoral positions at prestigious US research institutes, I finally opted to go to the National Institutes of Health in Bethesda, Maryland (under the mentorship of future Nobel Laureate Dr. Martin Rodbell) mainly because the NIH was one of the most prestigious research institutions in the US if not the world, and Marty was one of the most brilliant of a number of researchers there who were exploring the mechanisms of hormone action in the body. I thought by doing my training there that it would really jump-start my career as a scientist and I was absolutely right.

So it was that in February 14, 1981 (Valentines day and my daughter Karen's birthday) we all found ourselves on an Airplane heading for Washington DC to begin my three year post-doctoral fellowship at the NIH. The first days in the states were very challenging. Initially we lived in a room in the attic of Dr. Martin Rodbell's house and went apartment hunting on a daily basis. Eventually we found an apartment in Rockville Maryland. Marty had to co-sign my lease for the apartment as a guarantor because my NIH stipend (standard for foreign post-docs) only paid $13,000 per year in 1981. Suddenly I felt like a child again! Marty and his wife Barbara were very supportive helping us move and giving us a carpet for the apartment. After we bought some very cheap and nasty second hand furniture we were set up in our own place again.

Once settled, I found it fairly easy to fit into my new surroundings, as did my daughter, Karen, who attended the local school, but my wife Elaine never really liked living in the States and often wished she was back in the UK. It helped when she started to do some baby-sitting so she could keep busy during the day. Unfortunately, this was the only job that she could do since the JI visa that I had entered the US on had a restriction that the spouse of a visa holder was prohibited from working in the US. The next two years passed by quite uneventfully, my research was going well, despite the fact that my mentor Marty Rodbell left to go on a two year sabbatical in Geneva Switzerland shortly after my arrival at the NIH. My wife was now beginning to adjust to life in the US and my daughter was well established in the US school system. We even managed to buy a new car, a Chevette Scooter, which is essentially a stripped down Chevette with no air conditioning and plastic seats which gave you third degree burns in the hot humid brutal DC summers if you were foolish enough to sit on them wearing shorts! Life was good.

My NIH fellowship was extended for its final third year and during this time; I started to look around for other opportunities within the U.S. I had offers from Boston University and the University of California in

San Diego. No contest! After living in Washington for 3 years, I was ready to leave the East Coast and its hot humid summers and cold snowy winters, to me, San Diego represented a West Coast paradise, with temperate weather all year round! So in December 1983 we packed up our few belongings into a truck and drove our little Chevette across the US from Washington DC to San Diego. It took seven days of driving to get there, stopping at various locations along the way, including Knoxville in Tennessee, Little Rock in Arkansas, El Paso in Texas, Tucson in Arizona and finally San Diego in California. What a great trip, we saw a lot of the US with lots of interesting and diverse scenery. We stayed in the cheapest accommodations everywhere, usually a Motel 6. In San Diego, we quickly found an apartment in a community called Mira Mesa and we moved in the next day just in time before our furniture and belongings arrived from Washington DC.

Life in San Diego was wonderful; I loved the Hispanic culture and food. It was also a lot of fun to spend Christmas Eve on a beach by the Pacific Ocean over a nighttime campfire making "smores", heating marshmallow and a layer of chocolate between two graham crackers. My research at UC San Diego in the medical school also was going well and I continued to carry out research in the area of diabetes and the mechanism of action of insulin. We also used this time to travel and saw a lot of California over the next few years, traveling to Disneyland with our daughter, going to the desert to see the wild flowers bloom in Spring and enjoying the Beaches up and down the coast. Even the obligatory day trip to Tijuana, Mexico, was interesting, although the place itself seemed seedy and dirty, catering to all the worst excesses of what American tourists expected of a Mexican border town.

However, by mid 1984 my marriage was starting to crumble, my wife never really adapted to life in the

States and became increasingly unhappy, always comparing life in the States unfavorably to the life she had left behind in the UK. The constant negativity and unhappiness from her was sometimes difficult to cope with and I worked long hours at work to minimize having to deal with it. So it was against this background that I met the love of my life when I went back to the NIH for a 6-week spell in July 1984 to collaborate on a scientific project. The Post-Doc assigned to the project was a ravishingly beautiful woman from California, and I was immediately smitten by her charm, good looks, and intelligence. We worked together intensively on the project at the NIH for 6 weeks and I knew by the time that I left to fly back to California that I had met the person I wanted to spend the rest of my life with.

My wife and I divorced later that year and I flew back with her and my daughter as they returned to live in the UK. I wanted to make sure that they would be well settled. I was upset at the prospect of losing touch with my daughter Karen but decided that it would be best for both if she remained with my ex-wife. I had made the decision that I wanted to make my life in the States and this was in complete opposition with her strong desire to return to England. In retrospect, the divorce was probably the best in the long run for both of us. It took me many years to get over the guilt of what I had done, especially to my daughter, who I really cherished and loved a lot. Because of the emotional upheaval caused by this series of events, I always find it difficult to understand the way divorce is presented in the movies. Many films make light of the impact of divorce, when in reality it is not; it is full of years of anguish and guilt. I have found that the guilt never really leaves it just becomes quiescent for long periods of time and then resurfaces from time to time to inflict more pain.

On a positive note, my divorce was not too acrimonious and I remained on speaking terms with my ex-wife Elaine. She has never remarried and is living in my home town of Nottingham, where she is probably much happier than when she was living in the States. My daughter Karen is now very much grown up and is in her early 40's happily married with three children of her own, two boys and a girl. I have continued to stay in touch with Karen and visit her and my grandchildren whenever I travel to the UK to see my parents.

I left San Diego in March of 1985 and joined my old mentor Marty Rodbell who was now the Scientific Director of the National Institute of Environmental Health and Safety, NIEHS, an outpost of the NIH located in the Raleigh/Durham area of North Carolina. I found moving from San Diego to Raleigh North Carolina to be a culture shock for me. I moved to the East Coast to be closer to my future wife, who was still doing her post-doc at the NIH. While North Carolina was some distance from Washington, D.C, traveling time by car from Raleigh to Washington DC was a little over 4 hours, and I thought very doable. I frequently made the drive in my now well-worn Chevette.

In September 1986, we got married and we had a great honeymoon in Hawaii. I now had a stronger motivation to live closer to my new bride, who was now working as a faculty member at Rutgers University in New Jersey. Shortly thereafter, I got my first real job working as a Principal Scientist doing inflammation research at the DuPont Pharmaceutical Company in Glenolden Pennsylvania. We were finally in a position where we could actually begin a life together, albeit each with somewhat of a commute. We bought a house in Mount Laurel New Jersey, splitting our commutes; my wife had a 50 mile commute north on the New Jersey Turnpike, while I had a 35 mile trip south to Glenolden, which was just south of Philadelphia Airport. We were both excited to begin building a new life together in a beautiful home in South Jersey.

Life in South Jersey was interesting. One of the advantages was the proximity to Philadelphia. We both loved Philadelphia and would often drive in to the city to go to restaurants, movies or just hanging out on South Street. We explored the many historical sites of the site as well as ventured into the countryside. My wife became pregnant in January and we were blessed with a beautiful daughter in October 1987. This triggered a strong desire in both our hearts to live closer to family. Given my wife was born and raised in California and we both loved this state, we decided that it would be nice to move back to California and live near her family.

In the summer of 1989 we began exploring positions in the San Francisco Bay area and traveled west for multiple interviews. It proved to be quite a challenge to find two jobs in the same geographic location. By 1990, we decided to put our house in Mount Laurel up for sale so that if we managed to get a job offer on the West Coast we would be ready to move at a moments notice totally unencumbered. We also considered positions as far North as Seattle and as far South as San Diego. To keep our house "inspection ready", we needed to do some work to make the garden presentable as it was very woody and filled with lots of weeds. Because of this, we often had to do yard work, involving many hours of pulling weeds. Right before one trip out to California for an important job interview, I decided that I would go out and garden, even though I hated yard work, to improve the house's curb appeal. As we shall see in a moment this was one of the worst decisions I ever made.

Thus, it was on a really hot and humid July day that I found myself kneeling on the ground in the dirt by the side of my house pulling out weeds. The sun shone intensely and I was hot and sweaty, I really loathed gardening! Pre-occupied with my thoughts regarding the upcoming trip, the sale of the house and the prospect of the new job, I was startled by something small and dark that leapt out of the dirt and bit me on my exposed midriff while I was weeding. I had no idea what it was but decided to call it a day on the weeding! About one hour later I began to feel ill and began to develop a large red welt on my midriff. I felt so lousy that I decided to go to the doctor because I was worried I might not be able to travel. The doctor who examined the bite told me it was nothing and just to put an ice pack on the inflamed area to reduce the swelling.

Later that day, still feeling very ill, I flew out to join my wife in the San Francisco Bay Area where I had a job interview scheduled the following week. I boarded the flight, but found I spent most of the time in the bathroom of the plane putting cold compresses on my forehead and on the swelling on my midriff which was becoming even more red and inflamed. The flight to San Francisco seemed endless. I felt so ill, I was worried I would pass out. The Stewardesses were also very concerned for my well-being and constantly looked in on me. I arrived at San Francisco airport, was picked up, and fortunately was able to spend the next few days recovering in bed from whatever had bitten me. During that time, I continued to feel nauseated, ran a fever, and was only able to drink weak tea and other liquids. I was glad that we were staying with relatives and that I could totally focus on getting better.

After a long miserable weekend, I managed to muster enough energy to get out of bed and make myself presentable to go to my job interview at a

South San Francisco Biotech company called Genentech. Luckily the interview went well and I was able to focus on the science and not the residual pain/inflammation coming from my abdomen. After a few additional days of relaxing in the Bay Area with family we flew home. Despite my illness the trip had paid off since I got two job offers from Genentech in different departments and the rest of the summer passed by relatively uneventful.

In mid-September my parents flew over from England to stay with us and my wife's mother flew out from San Francisco as well. So we had a very full house. We went on day trips to Pennsylvania Dutch country and to the Jersey shore and our daughter Katherine got to spend some time with both sets of Grandparents, which she enjoyed tremendously. Then in late September I developed a really intense earache, often forcing me to spend the day in bed because of the pain. I went to the doctor several times and was prescribed multiple different antibiotics, however, none resolved the earache. After several weeks of this, I went to an ear nose and throat specialist, who told me I had a really red and inflamed eardrum and recommended that I have a myringotomy, which involves making a tiny incision in the eardrum, to relieve the pressure caused by the excessive build-up of fluid due to inflammation. I decided to have the procedure as I was fed up with the constant pain and the impact that it was having on my ability to do every day activities. The procedure was very painful and although I did have some immediate relief, after a couple of days I was back to the constant earache, and I returned to my regular physicians, and started with a complete check up, which included a chest x-ray, to see what the source of the problem could be. My physician was very concerned because my chest x-ray revealed numerous fluffy infiltrates in both of my lungs. The doctor referred to them as nodules, and all

I could think of was, don't let it be lung cancer. My doctor now prescribed a series of other tests, both because of the x-ray results but also because I had now developed very painful sinuses and a loss of appetite.

My wife and I were very concerned and worried about what was going on with my body. We were both frustrated by the multiple doctor's visits and lab tests, all leading to inconclusive results. Fortuitously, my wife, who was then working in the University of Medicine and Dentistry in New Jersey, happened to bump into one of the ear nose and throat specialists that we had seen early on in the process. She recounted my symptoms to him and he guided her to think about "diseases" that might present in the ear, although not specific to the ear, such as an autoimmune disease called Wegener's. She wrote down the name of this disease, which neither of us had ever heard of but would soon become very familiar with! By this time my doctors in Philadelphia had begun to come to the same conclusion. At the time, there were no definitive blood tests to support the diagnosis and they recommended admitting me to a hospital called Mercy Fitzgerald in Darby, Pennsylvania where they had attending rights, for some follow up tests. What followed was the start of my nightmares with Wegener's disease. I will continue with the story again in chapter 3, after I briefly describe the basis of the disease, its symptoms, diagnosis, prognosis and treatment in the next chapter.

Chapter 2   Wegener's Granulomatosis

As large and complex as humans are we are constantly under threat from tiny much less intricate micro-organisms, such as viruses, bacteria and protozoa, to which we become exposed during our lifetime. Successful invasion by these organisms can result in deadly and devastating diseases like polio, smallpox, AIDS, cholera, typhus, dysentery, malaria, etc. Some of these diseases like the plague (black death) in the Middle Ages have even changed the course of history by wiping out entire generations of individuals throughout Europe and Asia. Even more recently influenza epidemics like the Spanish flu outbreak in the early part of the twentieth century was almost as deadly as the plague, sickening and killing millions of individuals. To deal with this constant threat from these small but potentially deadly microbes, humans have developed a fairly robust defensive barrier known as the immune system. This has evolved over time to become a well-organized, efficient, killing machine, that can effectively eliminate and destroy most infectious agents that it encounters. Immune cells continually patrol the highways and byways of the human body in relentless pursuit of any pathogenic organisms that they encounter. Thus, although we are constantly exposed to these microbial invaders our highly evolved immune system usually enables us to resist being sickened by them.

Mostly this system of host defense works extremely well in protecting us from attack by pathogenic organisms. Sometimes, however, the host immune system can malfunction and turn upon itself damaging and killing its own tissues - this process of self-destruction is called autoimmunity. If it occurs in the joints rheumatoid arthritis can result, if the upper airways are attacked asthma ensues, if myelin in the central nervous system is damaged multiple sclerosis is the result. These and other diseases pose an ever-increasing health burden on our society and affect millions of individuals each year. Consequently pharmaceutical companies have poured billions of dollars into research and development to identify safe and effective drugs to treat these ailments and as a result an increasing repertoire of drugs are now available to treat these autoimmune diseases.

In contrast to the situation described above there are a number of autoimmune diseases that affect much smaller numbers of individuals but that can be equally, if not more, devastating. As a consequence these lesser known autoimmune diseases have not garnered as much attention from the pharmaceutical industry and thus their treatment options are less extensive than their more famous cousins. Amongst these there is a class of autoimmune diseases in which the immune cells attack the small blood vessels in the body. The ensuing inflammation and destruction that occurs is collectively known as vasculitis. These diseases have names that are not familiar to the general public but that are all too chillingly familiar to sufferers. They include microscopic polyangitis, Churg–Strauss syndrome, Kawasaki disease, Buerger's disease and Wegener's granulomatosis.

Wegener's granulomatosis, now more commonly known as granulomatosis with polyangiitis (GPA), is a potentially fatal vasculitis that mainly affects the small blood vessels of the sinuses, nose, throat, lungs and kidneys, but that can also involve the skin, eyes and other tissues. The initial symptoms of the disease depend on which organs or tissues are affected. More commonly it starts with painful and infected sinuses and chronic ear infections that do not really respond to treatment with antibiotics. Other symptoms are fatigue, fever, poor appetite and weight loss. If the lungs are involved the result is usually a cough that is often accompanied by shortness of breath. Left untreated, the disease can spread to other organs like the kidneys leading to organ failure and death.

Rapid advances in research have led to a clearer understanding of how the disease might be initiated. The culprits in this case are thought to be immune cells known as neutrophils which form the first line of defense against pathogens in what is called the innate immune response. Neutrophils are the most common type of white blood cell, or leukocyte, in the body and make up around 70% or so of our total immune cells. They kill pathogens by first engulfing them in a process known as phagocytosis. Once the neutrophils have taken up and enveloped the microbes they release a number of hydrolytic enzymes and free radicals that essentially punch holes into the microbes making them leaky and aiding in their digestion and total destruction. This whole process is often aided and abetted by the release of soluble immune factors such as complement and antibodies.

The hydrolytic enzymes in neutrophils are stored in granules inside the cytoplasm or cell interior. They are released once the neutrophil attaches and engulfs or surrounds what it considers to be a foreign cell or "non-self" by a process called degranulation. One of these granule proteins is an enzyme called proteinase-3 (PR-3), which is a serine protease. Proteases are enzymes that aid in the breakdown of proteins which are an important component of all living cells. PR-3 has a variety of physiological roles in host defense one of which includes the generation of an important immune defense molecule called interleukin-8. Interleukin-8 is a chemotactic agent, that belongs to a family of proteins called chemokines. These proteins are cellular chemoattractants that can summon immune cells like neutrophils from the circulation into tissues where they can become activated. Once activated, they can participate in fending off invasion by infectious agents. In addition, serine proteinases like PR-3 have been shown to be important in the generation of microbiocidal peptides (agents that kill or inhibit the growth of microbes), which can disrupt the normal cellular processes and metabolism of bacteria. PR-3 can also aid in the enzymatic degradation of the extracellular matrix and basement membrane proteins that surround cells making it easier for neutrophils to migrate through this cellular barrier to reach their target cells.

In summary then, neutrophils are very efficient at protecting us from invasion by pathogenic organisms, however, in GPA the normally protective neutrophils turn rogue and start attacking the very cells of the host organism that they normally protect. What is the basis for this destruction by friendly fire? To understand this we first have to understand the immune response in a little more detail. Recall that the innate immune response, in which neutrophils participate, is the first line of defense against infection, however, to overcome all of the strategies that microbes have developed over time to defeat this first line of defense we have evolved a second line of defense called the adaptive immune response. Put very simply the adaptive immune response enables the host to remember and recognize an attack by organisms that it has previously encountered. It involves cells known as T and B lymphocytes.

The adaptive immune response is also the basis for how vaccination works. When we are vaccinated we are immunized with either heat inactivated infectious agents or their toxins. These microbial proteins or foreign antigens then stimulate the B lymphocytes to generate antibodies against them. Much like a key that will only open the lock for which it was designed, these antibodies only recognize the specific antigen on the pathogenic organism that elicited their production. The antibodies are produced by the B lymphocytes in cooperation with the T lymphocytes. If we are exposed to these infectious agents again during our lifetime then these protective antibodies are rapidly released by B cells (that have remembered the infectious agent from their previous exposure to them) and participate in a number of processes to eliminate the pathogens or neutralize their toxins, thus protecting us from further infection. Immunization has been very successful in combating and eliminating a number of infectious diseases such as smallpox (totally eradicated) and polio (almost eradicated), which have been responsible for untold human misery and countless deaths over the centuries.

Interestingly it was noted in the early to mid 1980's that patients with GPA had high levels of an antibody, known as Anti Neutrophil Cytoplasmic Autoantibody (ANCA), in their cytoplasm. This antibody was initially detected in the serum of patients with rheumatoid arthritis and it was later found that the majority of patients with GPA also had high levels of ANCA. Research breakthroughs identified the neutrophil enzyme PR-3 as the major antigen responsible for ANCA production. As we have seen PR-3 is mainly stored in granules in neutrophils but in some otherwise normal individuals it can also be displayed on the cell surface through the plasma membrane. One theory to explain the generation of antibodies to a self-protein like PR-3 is by a process known as molecular mimicry. This is based on the idea that a microbial peptide generated during the destruction of infectious agents by immune cells might bear some homology or similarity to PR-3. The immune system sees this peptide as foreign and raises antibodies to it. These antibodies (ANCA) then recognize the PR-3 expressed on the surface of neutrophils and bind to them causing them to express more PR-3 antigens at the cell surface where they are available to bind more ANCA. The binding of ANCA to PR-3 on neutrophils induces the release of soluble factors like complement factors that through the alternative complement pathway stimulate the recruitment and activation of more neutrophils. Once activated the neutrophils release toxic factors, such as superoxide radicals and hydrogen peroxide, that cause inflammatory injury to the endothelial cells - the cells that line the walls of the blood vessels.

Once it was recognized that most GPA patients produce ANCA it was obvious that measuring the levels of these antibodies might aid in the diagnosis of the disease. GPA can initially be suspected in individuals who have complained of symptoms discussed earlier, such as constant ear ache, sinus and lung problems, etc. If follow up tests like x-rays showing immune infiltrates in the lungs, and urine tests that detect protein and red blood cells in the urine, together with blood tests that measure inflammation (sedimentation rate and C-reactive protein), are positive, then a specific blood test that assays for the presence of ANCA can be carried out. A positive ANCA assay, together with the symptoms described above, would strongly suggest that GPA is the cause. However, because the ANCA test was, in the early 1990's, only just emerging as a means of detecting GPA, physicians often liked to confirm their initial suspicions of the disease by carrying out a biopsy of inflamed and affected tissue to demonstrate the presence of granulomas (abnormal clusters of inflammatory cells). The granulomas are a strong indicator of the disease especially if they stain specific for the presence of ANCA.

Once the diagnosis of GPA was confirmed the treatment options for treating the disease in the early 1990's were pretty much the same for treating any autoimmune disease: Administer high doses of steroids known as glucocorticoids, to suppress inflammation, and infusions of a cellular poison known as cyclophosphamide (Cytoxan), which kills actively dividing cells such as immune cells.

Glucocorticoids belong to a large family of physiologically important molecules known as steroids. This family includes steroid hormones (sex steroids, anabolic steroids and glucocorticoids) as well as cholesterol. The major glucocorticoid produced by humans is called cortisol (hydrocortisone). Because glucocorticoids were shown to have important anti-inflammatory properties and were successfully used to treat rheumatoid arthritis in the 1950's a number of synthetic glucocorticoids that are pharmaceutically more potent than the endogenous molecules like cortisol have been synthesized as anti-inflammatory drugs by the Pharmaceutical industry. These synthetic glucocorticoids include dexamethasone, prednisolone and methyl prednisolone amongst others.

The steroids act by binding to specific receptors that are found on almost all cells of the body thus it might be anticipated that long-term use of high doses of steroids can have quite nasty side effects. In fact it turns out that they do. One of the side effects of long term glucocorticoid use are the effects on bone, resulting in an increased risk of osteoporosis and fractures. Glucocorticoids also have effects on metabolism and long-term use can result in hyperglycemia and diabetes. Since glucocorticoids act by suppressing the body's immune system it allows organisms that are normally kept in check to establish a foothold and set up opportunistic infections. These infections can rapidly proliferate and can be particularly devastating especially if they are in and around the mouth. Sometimes these infections become so severe that patients cannot eat properly and lose weight. As if this were not enough these hormones can also affect the brain and patients treated with high-dose steroids can become subject to mood swings, they can suffer from severe depression and they can become manic and display aggressive behaviors. All in all the side effects of treatment with high doses of steroids, although effective at reducing inflammation, can often come at a high cost to the patients.

Although steroids prolonged the average survival time for GPA patients, the major breakthrough in the treatment of the disease was the introduction of a drug called cyclophospamide (Cytoxan) in the early 1970's. Before Cytoxan was introduced, the mortality rate from GPA could be as high as 90% within one year, with the average survival being 5 months. Cytoxan is an organophosphate and is a first cousin of the mustard gas family that was used so effectively to poison soldiers in trench warfare during World War 1. Cytoxan was introduced in the late 1950's to treat a variety of tumors and it remains a cornerstone for the treatment of a variety of cancers to this day. It is part of the chemotherapy that helps to prolong the life of these patients. The drug acts by stopping the growth of actively dividing cells such as cancer cells. The success of cytoxan in treating autoimmune diseases like GPA came from the realization that since immune cells are also actively dividing cells if you block their growth with the drug you should have a beneficial effect by dampening down the immune response that initiates the cellular inflammation and damage. The drug works in treating GPA exactly as advertised. However, it is not too hard to imagine what the side effects of treatment with cytoxan might be, just ask any cancer patient who has undergone chemotherapy what their experience was like!

The most prominent side effects of cytoxan are: **thrombocytopenia** - which is a decrease in the number of platelets in the blood, leading to problems in wound healing because platelets play an important part in this process,

sterility - which can be quite problematic in young people and prevent them from starting a family,

leukopenia – which is a decrease in white blood cells and can, as discussed previously for steroids, lead to opportunistic infections,

severe Immuno-suppression – if the immune system is severely suppressed this can be life threatening if opportunistic microbes proliferate. This is similar to what AIDS patients, whose T lymphocytes have been wiped out by the human immunodeficiency virus (HIV-1), experience,

GI problems – the cells that line the intestinal gut are also rapidly dividing cells and cytoxan prevents their growth and replenishment inducing severe nausea and vomiting,

hair loss – many patients treated with cytoxan rapidly lose their bodily hair. This can be especially socially embarrassing for women who can become bald after treatment with the drug.

Thus, although treatment with steroids and cytoxan can be life saving, patients with GPA pay a high price in side effects when they are treated with these drugs. In fact some patients do quite poorly on this treatment because they cannot tolerate the side effects. It was clear then that new treatments for GPA that could replace cytoxan were badly needed and we will discuss this again in a later chapter. For now I would like to continue where I left off after the first chapter and describe what happened to me after I was admitted to hospital to diagnose and treat my suspected GPA.

Chapter 3 My Initial Battle With GPA

In October 1990 I was admitted to Mercy Fitzgerald Hospital in Darby, Pennsylvania with suspected GPA. Even though I had all of the signs and symptoms of the disease, including a positive ANCA test, the physicians there wanted to corroborate the diagnosis. I was told that the simplest way to confirm the disease was for them to perform a bronchoscopy which would enable them to take a tissue sample from my lungs. The sample would then be stained for the presence of granulomas. A bronchoscopy involves putting a bronchoscope, a flexible metal tube with a fiber optic camera, into the airways and lungs to visualize the areas for inflammation. Specimens can then be taken by biopsy for staining. I readily agreed to this procedure because I was feeling quite ill and just wanted the doctors to treat the illness and make it go away as rapidly as possible. After I had agreed to this procedure the doctors then told me that there was a good chance, however, that they might not be able to get the right piece of lung tissue to confirm my diagnosis and might have to do this repeatedly and that the procedure had some discomfort attached to it. They told me that a much better approach would be to do a lung biopsy under general anesthesia and that this had a higher chance of success than the bronchoscopy. They also told me that it was no big deal and that I would be released from the hospital within two weeks of the procedure. Because I was in a pretty depressed state of mind and just wanted to learn why I was ill I believed them and agreed to this procedure. This turned out to be an almost fatal mistake on my part.

First of all, a lung biopsy is a pretty involved procedure. After I was given a general anesthetic, the surgeon made a three inch incision in the skin of my chest just below my breast. Then they spread my ribs apart exposing my lungs. The surgeon then removed what he thought was a reasonable piece of tissue for staining of the suspected granuloma. After the biopsy the surgeon inserted a chest tube into the chest cavity to aid in the removal of air and/or fluid postoperatively.

I awoke from this procedure to what I can only describe as the worst pain I have ever experienced in my entire life. The surgeons had inserted a morphine drip that allowed me to self administer the drug to dull the pain, but even with the morphine the pain was so overwhelmingly intense that I almost could not stand it. I really cannot describe what it felt like other than I would rather die than go through it again! Within 24 hours of the operation and in constant pain, I now developed an infection. This shot my body temperature to 104°F and I was wracked in fevers and chills and transferred to the intensive care unit. My wife told me later that she was worried that I was going to die.

Somehow I survived the infection and it resolved slowly over the next couple of days. Now I just had the pain of the surgery and the extreme discomfort of the chest tube, which exacerbated the pain. I could not wait for them to remove it. They did this about 10 days after the operation. In the meantime I still had no appetite and was not eating. I started to develop bedsores from lying down all of the time. In addition, I was severely anemic with a hemoglobin level of 6 (a hemoglobin level of 13 to 17 is normal for a male) and I needed to be transfused with a couple of pints of blood. Then came the news from my doctors the biopsy was unsuccessful and I had gone through a near death experience for nothing! In the meantime they had started to treat me for GPA, with high dose steroids and cytoxan.

In my pretty poor medical state I did not tolerate the cytoxan at all, and I stopped taking it after a few days because I was so nauseous. The doctors replaced the cytoxan with a drug called Bactrim, an antibiotic, which is a combination of trimethoprim and sulfamethoxazole. This drug had been shown anecdotally to be potentially useful in some patients who had a mild form of GPA, like mine, which was mainly confined to the lungs and sinuses. In between the change of drugs and replacing the cytoxan with bactrim, I underwent another medical emergency and developed cardiovascular arrhythmia. The doctors were able to control this by using a cardiovascular drug called digoxin. In addition fluid was accumulating in my lungs and I was drowning in my own bodily fluids. For this the doctors prescribed a diuretic called furosemide (Lasix) that took care of this problem but that also resulted in hyperglycemia, a rapid increase in my blood sugar levels, as a side effect. Within a few weeks I had undergone major surgery and was being treated with a variety of drugs sometimes these were given in response to side effects from the drugs the physicians had initially treated me with!

Even with all of these treatments my physical condition had deteriorated quite rapidly during the time I had been in intensive care. My weight had dropped from 175 Ibs, which for a 6 foot one inch frame is normal, to around 140 Ibs. I was weak and not eating much because my medications made everything I tried to eat taste disgusting. I asked the doctors why this was but they had no ready answers. As I have since learned these symptoms can be partly attributed to the long term use of steroids. Many patients on long term steroids develop a fungal infection of the mouth which can also make everything you eat taste disgusting. Unfortunately for the patient most doctors do not really consider a loss of a sense of taste as an important medical problem and continue to treat the patient as before without too much concern. They are totally focused on treating the disease and sometimes lose sight of the mental state of the patient.

A combination of the surgery I had undergone together with my rapid weight loss left me feeling quite weak and I did not have enough strength or energy to get out of bed. A further consequence of being bed bound also left me severely constipated and I was feeling pretty low. I remember as I lay there thinking I would really like to switch places with the hospital janitor who was doing his menial labors in the hospital rooms but was upright, healthy and walking around. The statement made to me one night by one of the nurses doing her rounds did not further help my poor mental state. The nurse who took my vital signs and noted my poor medical condition told me "you should really consider transferring to a better hospital like Temple in Philadelphia to prevent your condition deteriorating even more "!

Despite my poor medical condition I made myself survive this experience because I had a family that really loved me and, my wife was also pregnant with our second child. I resolved to overcome everything that the illness could hurl at me and I concentrated on getting better so that my unborn child would get to know its father. So it was that after a couple of weeks that I was transferred to a unit of the hospital called telemetry. What I remember of my stay in this section of the hospital is that it was here that I learned to walk again, very slowly one or two feet at a time. I really felt like an invalid. I also recall the unit having flooding problems and not being able to get out of bed until they cleared the water away. One further delight that this hospital had in store for me!

Finally I was released from the hospital a few days before Thanksgiving. My thoughts were that I never wanted to go anywhere near that place again! I remember how good it felt to be home for Thanksgiving, and how our next-door neighbor's had lovingly prepared Thanksgiving dinner for us all. I wept with the sheer emotion of it and was glad to be alive and home again. Unfortunately within 10 days I was admitted to hospital again because I suddenly felt very ill, this time however it was probably not the GPA but a viral infection that laid me low. Based on my awful experience at Mercy Fitzgerald I admitted myself to Mount Holly Hospital in New Jersey where my daughter Katherine was born. This turned out to be a much better experience and I was released from the hospital feeling much better after a few days. During my stay I had a bout of very tarry bloody stools, which totally unnerved me, but they never returned again and I did not tell my doctors. After my horrible experience at Mercy Fitzgerald I wanted as few complications as possible.

In the next three weeks, I was well on the road to recovery. I was feeling well enough to pick up my parents from Philadelphia Airport. It was December 22nd and they had flown in from London to look after me and be with me over the Christmas period. The last time my mother saw me, I was extremely ill in a hospital bed. She had been extremely worried that I wouldn't survive so she was determined to fly back to the States again to visit me as soon as possible to make sure I was alright. You can imagine how surprised my parents were when I greeted them at the Airport. Apparently human resilience under severe medical duress is a force to be reckoned with. We all had a wonderful Christmas together, our first as a family for many years, and my mother cooked up a storm filling the fridge with enough meals to last a lifetime! My dad was busy too chopping enough wood from the forest at the back of our house to last us throughout the entire winter.

I spent the next three months building up strength again so that I could walk for more than a few steps at a time without feeling exhausted. I started back at work at Dupont in mid-January and by March I was almost fully recovered from the illness. So it was that in early April, my wife and daughter and I moved from our home in Mount Laurel, New Jersey to San Mateo in California where my wife and I both started positions at a biotechnology company called Genentech. My wife was in the development side of the company and I was in the research side. What a crazy year we had been through. I remember noting in the Christmas letter that we sent out that year – "Nothing much happened this year, one of us recovered from a near death experience, we sold our house in New Jersey, we quit our jobs, we relocated almost 3000 miles away in California, we started new jobs at Genentech, we had a baby boy and we bought a new house in the San Francisco Bay Area" - altogether a pretty standard year!

All in all, I still had to cope with the fact that I had contracted an uncommon disease. GPA is a rare disease that affects only about 30 people per million thus there are probably only around 10,000 patients with the disease in the United States. How was it then that I managed to be unlucky enough to get the disease given these odds. Was Lady Luck against me or are there some reasonable scientific explanations to account for this?

Chapter 4   How Did I Get GPA – some ideas

As we have already seen the immune system can be both our friend and our deadliest enemy. We would not survive very long in the absence of a strong host defense mechanism. Not only are we constantly assailed by microorganisms in the air that we breathe, but also those that permeate into almost every aspect of our environment. In fact there are individuals who are born with a genetic disorder known as SCID (Severe combined immunodeficiency) who have an almost totally impaired immune system. These individuals (typified by Tod Lubitch whose life was portrayed in the movie "the boy in the bubble" and who lived in a plastic bubble for many years) quickly succumb to infections that most of us can simply shrug off because of our robust immune system. The immune system is pretty sophisticated because it has learned how to recognize foreign invaders that can harm us but in general it does not usually attack its own tissues. This process is known as discriminating between self and non-self. It is also part of the reason that tissue transplants are quickly rejected because they are recognized by the immune system as foreign. To prevent this tissue rejection transplant patients are given strong immuno- suppressive drugs like cyclosporine which dampen the immune system and allow the transplanted organ to survive.

So given this tightly regulated system of control why then did my immune system turn rogue and start attacking its own tissues? There are at least two reasons to account for this, the first is quite likely associated with my genetic makeup and the second is probably associated with the insect bite that I described in the first chapter. Lets examine each in turn, first the genetic factors. As humans we are all genetically distinct and this includes our immune cells. These cells are tagged with a family of molecules called the **M**ajor **H**istocompatability **C**omplex proteins or MHC. The MHC proteins are responsible for presenting bits of foreign antigen (from microbes that have been destroyed by the immune cells) to T cells and other immune cells to activate them. This is analogous to a bloodhound sniffing clothing from an escaped prisoner and then tracking him down based on the unique smell. For example each of the antigens presented is unique and it leads to the activation of a particular set of immune cells. If these microbes are never encountered again during the life of the host then these immune cells remain quiet. However if these same microbes are encountered by the host again then these specific immune cells will sniff them out and initiate an attack against them destroying them and protecting the host.

Humans can express a variety of MHC proteins on their immune cells and some of these have been linked or associated with a propensity to autoimmune disease. For example expression of the DR3 type is associated with an almost 5-fold increase in the risk of getting multiple sclerosis, expression of the DR2 type is associated with a 15-fold increase in the risk of developing a particular nasty autoimmune disease called Goodpasture's syndrome, which destroys the kidneys. These risk factors do not mean that individuals expressing these MHC molecules will get these diseases it just means that it increases their risk of getting them compared to individuals who do not express them. This is analogous to the increased risks of cardiovascular disease and certain cancers in individuals who are overweight, smoke and lead a sedentary life.

Now even before I developed GPA I had another autoimmune disease called vitiligo and unlike GPA it is non-life threatening. In vitiligo the cells that produce the melanin in the skin that protects us against the harmful effects of the ultraviolet rays from the sun, stop making melanin and there is a loss of skin pigment. This can have consequences if affected individual's stay out in the sun too long since it can lead to severe sun-burns and long term even skin cancer or melanoma. Because of the vitiligo my normal tan colored skin has patches that are quite pale. This can be quite disfiguring in individuals with very dark or black skin. I have however learned to live with it and take appropriate precautions when I go out I the sun. The reason that I am sharing that I have vitiligo is to point out that this autoimmune disease also has been shown to be associated with the expression of certain types of MHC molecules and it raises the idea that my genetics are such that if I encounter the right set of circumstances my immune system will react in a certain way that might predispose me to autoimmunity. In contrast, individuals with a different set of MHC proteins encountering the same circumstances that triggered my autoimmunity may remain totally unaffected by this and not develop any autoimmune disease.

So what were the specific set of circumstances that, given my unique MHC genetics, could have triggered my immune cells to inappropriately attack their own tissues? Well remember the insect bite that started all of this off. In most people an insect bite is harmless and other than itching and redness, usually due to the injection of bacteria into the wound, has no long lasting consequences. In my case though, I felt really sick for several days after I had been bitten. This was probably due to an allergic reaction. Recall that microbial invasion into the body induces a very robust immune reaction to destroy the bacteria. When the bacteria are destroyed, usually by the bodies first line of defense (neutrophils and macrophages), bits of the dead bacteria are presented by the MHC molecules to arm T lymphocytes to recognize the bacteria if they try to invade again in the future. Sometimes the bits of bacterial proteins that are presented by the MHC molecules can bear a strong molecular resemblance to some of the proteins that we produce (host proteins) and the immune machinery now swings into action to activate T cells and produce antibodies against self (the host proteins) leading to autoimmunity. This process is called molecular mimicry.

It was possible that the robust immune response to the bacterial infection from my insect bite resulted in the destruction of the microbes by neutrophils and macrophages. Recall from above that these cells are programmed to engulf and destroy any invading bacteria. If one of the pieces of bacterial protein produced from this immune response resembled the PR3 molecules exposed on the surface of my neutrophils this would, by the process of molecular mimicry, induce the production of antibodies to this self protein. Thus, the next time I got an infection and my neutrophils were activated, the antibodies to PR3 produced by the activated B cells would react with the membrane bound PR3 on the surface of my neutrophils, aggregating and activating them, as described earlier, to initiate an immune attack against my own cells. This scenario might also explain why the antibiotic bactrim that I was given when I first contracted GPA worked so well, in tandem with the steroids, to combat the disease. The antibiotic would act to kill the bacteria thus perhaps not producing such an exuberant immune response by the neutrophils and therefore limiting the severity of the autoimmune attack on my cells. All of this is of course mere speculation, as my doctors were quick to point out when I discussed it with them. However, they certainly had no alternative explanations for what suddenly precipitated the disease and in fact I detected that they were not really interested either. As a scientist and a patient I find this lack of curiosity really short-sighted. It is obvious that every piece of critical information that we can glean about what causes GPA can be potentially useful for research scientists to help to design better drugs to target this disease much more effectively in affected individuals. As we have seen it is not as if we have a wonderful arsenal of drugs to treat GPA, and better more effective drugs with less side effects would be gratefully received by the patients. In fact there are now some much better drugs than cytoxan to treat GPA and I will expand on this in a later chapter.

Chapter 5   The Intervening Years

Lets restart the narrative of my battle against GPA where I left it at the end of chapter 3. It is now May 1991, my wife and I had started new jobs at Genentech and we had a new addition to the family, our son Christopher. One of the first things I did when we arrived in California was to find a doctor who was familiar in treating patients with GPA. Here I really lucked out because the doctor who was recommended to me was Dr. Elaine Lambert, a rheumatologist at Stanford Hospital. She has proven to be a superb clinician with a very caring attitude to her patients. She is always available no matter how trivial the problem and has been my physician through thick and thin for over 24 years now. But I am getting a little ahead of myself. When I went for my first consultation with Dr. Lambert I was still being weaned down slowly on steroids and she recommended adding a drug called methotrexate which acts by suppressing the activation of T lymphocytes and thus is helpful in treating autoimmune diseases such as rheumatoid arthritis and GPA in which these cells play a role. Over the next few months I came off the steroids completely and was being maintained on the methotrexate. Initially, I had lab tests done every 3 months, and later, every six months. The major test was always the ANCA assay, which was becoming more and more accepted by doctors as a diagnostic for detecting active disease in GPA patients. Although it is certainly true that not all GPA patients have an increase in ANCA levels when the disease is active, many including myself do. Thus for me the ANCA was always a pretty good predictor of the state of my disease.

Over the next couple of years my ANCA levels were checked and apart from a few slightly positive readings most were negative and I had no symptoms other than the constant sinus inflammation. In 1994 I moved from Genentech to join another West Coast Biotechnology company called Berlex Biosciences (based in Richmond California), which was the American subsidiary of a German Pharmaceutical company called Schering AG. We lived in a house in a Bay Area city called Belmont which meant that my wife only had a short 20 min commute to work in South San Francisco, while I had a much more challenging 50 min commute which included having to cross the Bay Bridge. In addition my job involved travelling to my companies headquarters in Berlin, Germany, sometimes as much as 8 times a year. This obviously increased my stress levels, which is never a good thing especially when you have an autoimmune disease like GPA. In 1995 I was a speaker at a scientific meeting in Bath England. At the end of my seminar one of the attendees who was a pulmonary specialist came up to me acting quite concerned and told me that he was worried by the apparent stridor that he detected in my voice during my seminar. He explained that stridor, which is a high pitched wheezing sound, usually occurs as a result of a narrow or obstructed airway and that I should go to a pulmonologist and have it checked out immediately upon my return to the States. Interestingly on my last visit to my doctor I had complained that I was experiencing some breathing difficulties, I am a lap swimmer and it had become increasingly more difficult to swim because I was always breathless.

Following this advice I went back to my doctor and she sent me to an ear, nose, and throat specialist at Stanford. My examination included a microscopic direct laryngoscopy which involved passing a very thin flexible tube with a fiber optic camera through my nose and down into the larynx so that the vocal chords and glottis could be visualized. Although I felt like gagging during this procedure it was all over in a couple of minutes with no ill effects. The doctor told me that I had subglottic stenosis, a narrowing of the airway or larynx (which is below the glottis or vocal chords), which, if it is severely occluded, can be a life-threatening airway emergency. My airway was about 60 to 70% occluded and he recommended that I have a procedure called microscopic laser direct laryngoscopy in which a laser is used to open up the airways. He assured me that it was only a minor operation, takes about 30 minutes or so and is carried out under general anesthesia, and that I would feel much better after the procedure with little if any ill-effects. I agreed to this and with some trepidation found myself in an operating room at Stanford towards the end of 1995. The doctor was absolutely right I woke up from the operation with a slightly sore throat but no other problems. After an overnight stay I went home the next day and my breathing was now much less labored than before, what a difference! The airway occlusion that I experienced is common in GPA patients with upper airway involvement and is probably due to a build up of the fibrotic tissue and the granulomas that are so typical of the disease. I was lucky that mine was detected and excised before it got so bad that it could be life threatening. Patients with GPA have been known to die from upper airway obstruction so it is important to have it evaluated by a specialist. Over the next 17 years I had at least 5 more laser procedures, about every two years or so. Then the doctors switched to simply dilating the airway (stretching it with a medical instrument that is inserted into the airway) and carrying this out by swabbing the area with a drug called mitomycin. This drug inhibits the growth of fibroblasts that cause the fibrosis and contribute to the narrowing of the airway. With this procedure my airways have become less constricted and I have had fewer procedures over the intervening years, which is an obvious advantage.

The years passed by quite pleasantly and my health was pretty good, apart from the occasional dilation laryngoscopies, my GPA seemed to be under control and my ANCA levels were usually negative. Life was pretty good, then in 2006 Schering AG was acquired by another German company called Bayer AG (who are most well known as producers of aspirin) who promptly decided to close down Berlex and lay-off most of its employees including me. This was pretty shocking because I had not seen it coming and thus was not prepared for it. They say that the three most stressful events in life are losing a loved one, getting divorced and losing your job. Now I was facing one of those three. However, the termination package that I got from Berlex was pretty good and I received full pay and bonus for the next 18 months, which almost saw me through to the end of 2008.

During my period of unemployment I made the most of my social life, swimming almost daily, meeting with friends for drinks and generally enjoying life. It was also during this period that my friend Sofia and I decided to form a small company. We called it Jararaca Bio and it was based around peptides isolated from the South American pit viper Bothrops jararaca which had been shown to have anti-hypertensive effects, amongst others, and which had led to one of the major marketed drugs to treat high blood pressure, the ACE inhibitor Captopril.

Sofia and I pursued this venture vigorously and made several pitches to investors. Unfortunately because of the early nature of this potential product we were not successful in getting funding to pursue the program any further. Nevertheless I had fun doing this especially since our third partner a well known Brazilian scientist invited us to Sao Paulo in Brazil to present a seminar at his institute and meet with his scientists who had gathered some early data on this project. I enjoyed my trip to Brazil tremendously visiting Rio de Janeiro where I drank Caiparinhas and barbequed meats on the beautiful beaches, all in all I had a blast. I searched for the Girl from Ipanema in vain!

However, all good things have to come to an end sometime and by the end of 2008 I had managed to find a position at UC Davis at the medical school in Sacramento. I was hired as an academic coordinator and visiting professor to help in teaching pharmacology to 1st and 2nd year medical students. In addition I taught drug discovery to post graduate students at the Davis campus. I enjoyed this tremendously, except for the fact that I was driving to Sacramento every day, a 75-minute commute each way. After a year of this, the commuting was starting to wear me down so I was somewhat relieved when in the summer of 2010 my contract at UC Davis was not renewed. At this point I decided I would continue at UC Davis as a clinical faculty volunteer delivering several lectures *pro bono* and retiring from full time work to enjoy my life.

In 2011 we were planning a holiday in Portugal with our close friend, Sofia, who was Portuguese. Debbie and I had visited in Portugal earlier that year in January and fell in love with the food, the wine, the country and its people. There was something about the Portuguese Fado and culture that struck a chord with me and I couldn't wait to go back there in the summer. However, it was in April of 2011 that I started to feel like I was fighting off a chest infection. I was feeling tired and listless and had this horrible hacking cough that I couldn't get rid of. I saw both my rheumatologist and a pulmonologist and had a bunch of lab tests done including an ANCA which was negative. The pulmonologist gave me an inhaler that included a bronchodilating agent to open up my airways and a steroid to reduce any inflammation. I ambled along with this until mid-May and then went back again to visit my pulmonologist. My usual physician was on vacation and her partner sent me for a chest x-ray, which was clear, and put me on a low dose of steroids, 10 mg per day which was titred down over the next few weeks to zero. This appeared to help so that in late June I decided that I would be fine to travel to Portugal. As it turned out this was another major mistake that was going to cost me dearly.

Chapter 6 An Old Nemesis Returns

My wife and I boarded our United Airlines flight to London at San Francisco International Airport on June 24 around 1 pm and arrived at Heathrow the next day at 7 am. It was, as usual, a long and tiring flight and we were both exhausted even though we traveled in the business section. We had a layover in London for a few hours, and then flew on a British Airways flight landing in Lisbon around 1pm. Our friends Don and Sofia and their daughter Patricia were at the airport in Lisbon to meet us. Sofia had arranged for us to stay at a variety of farmhouses or Quintas for the next 10 days and we were looking forward to it. After dropping off our luggage at her parent's house where we were spending our first night we drove into a suburb of Lisbon called Belém to stop at a pastry shop to eat the local pastries called Pastéis de Belém. They are a sort of creamy custard cup wrapped in a flaky quite delicious pastry. I had become addicted to them on my previous trip and Sofia knowing this had arranged for us to go there as a treat. Some excellent Port, that the Portuguese are famous for, accompanied the pastries. The only thing that spoiled this most perfect of days was that my hacking cough was back and slowly starting to get worse. Thus it was that we stopped off in the town to buy some cough medicine to try to suppress the cough. That evening we accompanied Sofia's parents to a barbeque in aid of the local scouts. It was a nice evening the people we met including Sofia's brother-in- law and sister were very friendly and nice. However as the evening wore on, and despite the cough medicine, my cough just would not subside and it was starting to make my ribs ache. I started not to feel so great, so after a couple of hours my wife Debbie, Sofia, her mother and I went back to her house and Debbie and I went to our room for the evening. I remember thinking how hot it was;

Lisbon in June can get up to 90°F and be quite humid thus we slept with the window open to catch any breeze that was out there. But to no avail the air was very still and all we caught with the window open was the noise from the urban neighborhood, which made it quite difficult to sleep. The next morning I awoke after sleeping for a few hours, I was jet lagged, and tired from all of the coughing, but nevertheless looking forward to driving to our first Quinta, which was about a couple hours north of Lisbon. We had rented a minivan since there were five of us, Sofia, her husband Don, their daughter Patricia, my wife Debbie, and I, and all of our associated luggage and belongings. On the way to the farmhouse we stopped briefly at Sofia's parent's farm, which was just north of Lisbon and said hello to her sister and brother-in-law who were staying in one of the houses on the property. We drove further north and spent the first of two nights at Quinta do Troviscal close to the town of Tomar.

The farmhouse was really nice with a garden setting and a pool overlooking a local river. The rooms were small but clean and quite pleasant. That evening I started to feel really ill. I was tired but could not sleep. My heart was pounding, and my cough was getting worse and I was short of breath and felt really listless. We had breakfast served on our terrace in the morning and I concentrated on trying to feel better because I really did not want to spoil the vacation for all of the others. By around 11am however it was apparent to Debbie that I was really not feeling very well and she and Sofia drove me to the emergency room in the town of Tomar. Thank goodness that Sofia was there since she was able to communicate with the doctors and staff on my behalf. I got an x-ray and blood work done and the doctor examined me and told me that I had atrial flutter. An atrial flutter is an abnormal heart rhythm that is usually associated with a fast heart rate. In some cases it can lead to atrial fibrillation with an increased risk of strokes. He gave me some medication, Amiodarone, to control the flutter and told me that my chest x-ray was clear and that I had no infections. My total stay in the emergency room barely lasted 4 hours but the suffering that I saw there will stay with me for a lifetime!

The cough medicine that I was taking was next to useless since it had no effect on suppressing my cough, so I threw it away and toughed it out. We left the Quinta and headed north the following day to a small village east of Coimbra about 250 km north of Lisbon. We stayed at Quinta de Alem do Ribeiro which had beautiful gardens, nice bedrooms, and a pool with deck chairs and loungers for relaxing in. I was still feeling pretty tired so I spent most of my time lying by the pool reading a book. The others went on a walk near the town and picked me up a little bit later and I joined them in a shady spot by the river where we had a small snack and some drinks. A really pleasant way to spend the day. The dinners in the evening at the farmhouse were excellent, so good in fact that Sofia's husband Don could not stop eating! After two days at the farmhouse I still felt pretty listless and not my usual exuberant self. It was hard for the others not to notice my depressed state and I felt conscious that I was probably ruining the vacation for everyone and I wished I were back home so that they would not have to deal with it.

We left two days later heading northeast to our destination Casas de Pousadouro near Baiao, which was about 90 km east of Porto on the Douro River. This farmhouse was a real jewel with absolutely spectacular scenery on a hill overlooking the Douro where some of the best wines in Portugal, and indeed Europe, are produced. The accommodation was first class and just seeing this place lifted my spirits up.

How I wished that we had spent all of our vacation there. We stayed there for four days and were joined there by Sofia's parents, her sister and brother-in-law and their two children. They were there to celebrate Sofia's sisters 50th birthday and we were happy just to be there and join in the celebrations. The farmhouse had kayaks for paddling on the river and also a nice swimming pool and a large spacious deck for just lolling around on. I read my book and really enjoyed the views of the Douro valley and the river down below. There was even a single-track railway line, which crossed a narrow bridge over the river, and it was very relaxing just to lie on a lounger and watch life passing by. The next three days passed quite quickly and during our stay there we had the chance to cruise down the Douro on a small boat where we saw some beautiful homes and gardens and plenty of vineyards on both sides of the river. The boat ride was followed by lunch of some freshly caught fish at a small local restaurant by the side of the river.

It was time to drive to our final destination a small resort hotel south of the Douro and on the way back to Lisbon. This was a very different experience from our peaceful farmhouse on the banks of the Douro. The hotel was noisy, it had a number of outdoor swimming pools and a poolside bar, but remarkably had closed its kitchens down for the days we were there so that we had to drive to a local restaurant, which was good, for dinner. The poolside bar served snacks during the day and everyone had fun during the day drinking caipirinhas and eating hamburgers and fries. I was really trying to join in the fun and put on what I thought was a positive facade during the day. At night lying there in my bed, I just tried to focus on feeling positive even though with every fiber of my being I just felt really lousy. During our stay at the hotel we phoned my doctor in the States and arranged for me to see her as soon as I arrived back home.

I remember the flight home being really difficult. I was feeling really ill and was wheeled from Lisbon Airport in a wheelchair to the plane. Debbie and I flew from Lisbon to London and spent the night in a really luxurious airport hotel in Terminal 5. Neither of us cared about the expense it did not really seem to matter set against the backdrop of my ill health. I was really concentrating on surviving the long 10-hour journey back to the States the next day. Somehow the journey passed by and we landed in San Francisco on Friday July 8th, I was never happier to be back in my home than now. On the following Monday I saw my doctor and she was appalled by my poor physical state. She told me that she suspected that the GPA had returned and she set me up for three intravenous infusions of 500 mg of steroids daily over the next three days. This was primarily to really ramp down the inflammation, which by now was really obvious. I also had a blood chemistry done later that week at John Muir Medical so that my ANCA and various other parameters could be assessed. My doctor also told me that a new treatment had just been approved to treat GPA, a drug called Rituxan marketed by Genentech. This drug offered renewed hope for patients who had been battling the disease at the expense of some potentially nasty side effects with the currently available treatments. I think it will be instructive at this point to break into my narrative and discuss the science behind the approval of Rituxan for treating GPA.

Chapter 7 Rituxan - A New Treatment for GPA

Rituxan is a drug that was developed and approved to treat various cancers including non-Hodgkins lymphoma (NHL). This blood cancer results in the unrestricted growth of a form of white blood cells that we have already met, the B-lymphocytes. The end result is the formation of solid tumors called lymphomas that if left untreated, lead to death. Rituxan is an antibody that recognizes and binds to a protein antigen called CD20 that decorates the surface of these B-lymphocytes. It probably works by marking the cells that it binds to for destruction by a variety of immune-mechanisms and it has been very successful in treating these and other white blood cell cancers. A similar mechanism probably lies at the core of the success of Rituxan in treating GPA. As we discussed earlier the driving force for the destruction wreaked by the neutrophils on the endothelial cells that line small blood vessels is probably fueled by the production of ANCA by the B-lymphocytes. So if we can destroy these B-lymphocytes with Rituxan it should be beneficial in the treatment of GPA. This was the reasoning behind a study that had been published in 2010 in a premiere Medical Journal called the New England Journal of Medicine. This study paved the way for the approval of Rituxan for the treatment of GPA.

In this study patients were treated with high dose glucocorticoids in combination with either Rituxan or Cytoxan in multicenter clinical trials. Clinical trials are carried out to test whether drugs that are proposed to treat disease are effective and safe. Typically drugs have to successfully negotiate three separate levels of clinical trials called phase I, II and III before they are approved for clinical use in patients. In the United States this approval is granted by a government agency called the Food and Drug Administration or FDA.

The study compared Rituxan and Cytoxan in treating 197 ANCA positive patients who had either GPA or polyangiitis (another inflammatory disease of the small blood vessels). The 99 patients in the Rituxan group received the drug by intravenous infusion once a week for four weeks while the 98 patients in the control group received Cytoxan once daily. Both treatment groups received one to three pulses of high dose glucocorticoids to ramp down inflammation, followed by a regimen of much lower doses of steroids that were eventually tapered down to zero over the course of the next five months for patients who responded to the treatment. The measure of the success of the treatment, clinically known as the primary end point, was the complete remission of active disease. This was defined by a **B**irmingham **V**asculitis **A**ctivity **S**core (BVAS) of zero. The BVAS measures disease activity in GPA patients based on a variety of parameters (renal, cardiovascular, pulmonary, etc) that examine whether a patient either has symptoms of persistent disease or whether the patient has new or worsening disease. For example renal involvement would include measuring creatinine levels, hypertension, proteinuria, haematuria all of which are good indicators of how well the kidneys are functioning.

Sixty-three of the patients in the Rituxan group (64%) reached the primary end point compared with 52 in the control group (53%). Analysis using a variety of statistical methods showed that these differences in response in the two treatment groups were not significant. In simple terms the Rituxan therapy was as effective as the Cytoxan treatment for inducing remission in severe disease. Even more encouraging was the finding that a greater percentage of patients in the Rituxan group who had relapsing disease reached the primary endpoint compared with those receiving Cytoxan. These results indicated that Rituxan could be superior to Cytoxan in the treatment of the relapsing disease.

As discussed earlier the major impetus for finding new therapies with which to treat GPA patients was to find safer drugs with fewer side effects than the current therapy of Cytoxan. It was clear from this study that Rituxan appeared to be better tolerated by patients than Cytoxan. For example more patients in the Cytoxan group had one or more of the predefined selected adverse events. This included more episodes of leukopenia; a fall in the number of white blood cells that can, as discussed earlier, lead to increases in infection. As a final note, although not mentioned in the study, it would have been instructive to canvass patients for side effects such as nausea and vomiting, stomach ache, diarrhea, etc, all of which are common side effects of Cytoxan treatment, to determine whether there were differences in the two groups of patients.

The history of the development of Rituxan is instructive in helping to understand why it takes so long to find new therapies for the treatment of disease. The development of Rituxan started at a small biotechnology company called IDEC in the early 1990s. The idea was to use selective therapies to destroy cancer cells rather than the non-selective approaches such as chemotherapy and radiation, which not only killed cancer cells but also killed normal cells and were very unpleasant for the patients undergoing therapy. Sometimes the treatment became so intolerable for some patients that they chose to die rather than go through another grueling round of treatment. Clearly more selective treatments that only killed cancerous cells and not normal cells were required. One way to achieve this was to determine what made cancer cells different from normal cells and to design a "magic bullet" to selectively destroy them. As we have already discussed B-lymphocytes, which can become malignant and cause lymphomas, express a cell surface protein called CD20. Most other cells in the body do not express this protein and so if we can selectively kill cells through targeting CD20 only B-lymphocytes will be affected. This idea formed the basis behind the approach of treating B cell lymphomas at IDEC.

To effectively target cells expressing CD20 the approach at IDEC was to generate monoclonal antibodies against the protein. Monoclonal antibodies are proteins made by a single immune cell and differ from polyclonal antibodies which are produced by a variety of immune cells. Monoclonal antibodies thus offer the advantage of producing proteins that are identical in how they recognize a specific target protein or antigen, in contrast to polyclonal antibodies which can bind to different areas of the target protein. Monoclonal antibodies against a specific protein or antigen are produced by immunizing a mouse with the protein of interest and then harvesting the B-lymphocytes from the mouse spleen. These cells will include B-cells against the antigen. These B-cells are then made immortal by fusing them with a human myeloma, a form of cancer cell, and those cells that are specific for the antigen are then selected in specific media. With this technology a variety of different monoclonal antibodies that recognize different epitopes (an epitope is a specific antigenic region of a protein) of an antigen can be generated. These antibodies can be useful therapeutically because they can be designed specifically to only target a certain antigen, such as one that is found on cancer cells.

The first monoclonals against CD20 were produced at IDEC in 1991 and after successfully filing an IND (Investigational New Drug Application) in

1992 with the FDA to allow the drug to be used in clinical trials, IDEC formed a collaboration in 1995 with another biotechnology company called Genentech to co-develop the drug for cancer indications. The drug was finally approved for NHL in 1997 and because it depletes CD20 B cells, which as we have seen are an important part of the immune system, clinicians began investigating Rituxan in autoimmune diseases such as rheumatoid arthritis and multiple sclerosis. This led to the approval of Rituxan, when used in combination with methotrexate, for the treatment of patients with rheumatoid arthritis. As we have already seen, Rituxan was approved for the treatment of patients with GPA in 2010. Its approval took more than twenty years of intense preclinical and clinical research, probably involving hundreds of millions of dollars, for the drug to be approved. This is part of the reason why the discovery of new drugs is sometimes such a slow and tortuous process.

An interesting aside before we continue. While I was working at Berlex in 1997 a colleague of mine moved to a biotechnology company called Coulter Pharmaceutical (later acquired by Corixa) which was very interested in monoclonal antibody approaches targeting various cancers. The company was specially interested in CD20 approaches and one of its major competitors was of course IDEC pharmaceuticals. At this time I was intrigued by the progress that IDEC was making in this arena and started buying stock in the company. By the time that IDEC was acquired by Biogen, I had made a nice return on my original investment in the stock market. So it is somewhat ironical that Rituxan not only benefited me financially but also clinically.

Chapter 8 An Old Nemesis Returns Continued

About a week after having my blood work done after I returned from Portugal, I got my test results back. The results made pretty dismal reading; not only was my ANCA assay strongly positive but my PR3 levels were sky high at 750, levels of less than 10 were considered negative. In addition, my C-reactive protein (CRP) which is a protein produced by the liver during the acute phase of inflammation, and is thus used as a measure of inflammation, was 189, less than 10 is normal. My kidneys also were damaged because the creatinine levels and glomerular filtration rate (GFR) which are used to assess kidney function were high and low respectively. Kidney damage was further indicated by the presence of protein in the urine, which should be absent in normally functioning kidneys, and by the presence of casts, and red blood cells. Furthermore my hemoglobin was low, as was my hematocrit. The kidney produces a protein called Epogen that regulates the levels of red blood cells, and damaged kidneys obviously have an impaired ability to produce red blood cells resulting in low hemoglobin and hematocrit which give rise to anemia. My symptoms together with the clinical tests suggested I was in the full throes of a major relapse of my disease which had returned with a vengeance after almost 20 years of remission. As if all of this was not enough the atrial flutter that I was experiencing in Portugal had now turned into atrial fibrillation. A few years previously I had undergone a procedure known as a catheter ablation which can be used to treat some forms of arrhythmia including atrial flutter. The procedure involves inserting a catheter, which is a thin, flexible wire, into the femoral vein which is in the groin. The catheter is then guided into the heart through the blood vessel. High frequency electrical impulses are then used to destroy any area of the heart tissue where abnormal heartbeats may cause an arrhythmia to start. This treatment had been quite successful for me previously in treating my atrial flutter. My cardiologist told me that I could have the same procedure to treat the atrial fibrillation. It was a little riskier but had a good chance of success. I opted for the treatment since the fibrillation was making me feel really tired and on top of the GPA was too much to deal with.

In the meantime my doctor prescribed Rituxan infusions once a week for four weeks at Stanford. The infusions involved a pre-infusion of 500 mg of steroids and some Benadryl which is an anti-histamine and is used to dampen down any allergic reactions to the infusion which can occur. Reading the little information booklet about Rituxan is pretty scary because of course it lists all of the side effects that can occur. The most serious ones are infusion reactions, and PML (progressive multifocal leukoencephalopathy) which is a rare, serious brain infection which can lead to death. The infusion reactions seem to occur mostly when patients are given intravenous doses of monoclonal antibodies of any sort, like Rituxan, and the symptoms are not very pleasant. They can include hives or rash, itching, swelling of the lips, tongue, throat, or face, a sudden cough, shortness of breath, difficulty breathing, dizziness, and heart palpitations and chest pain. PML is caused by a virus which is found in most people without inducing any medical problems. But if the immune system is weakened in any way, for example by taking immunosuppressive drugs, then the virus can infect the brain and PML can develop. In fact a number of patients with multiple sclerosis who have been treated with another monoclonal antibody called Tysabri have developed PML and died. This actually caused Tysabri to be withdrawn from the market because of these risks, but patient pressure forced it back onto the market where it now carries a black box warning.

So with all of these potential side effects it was with some trepidation that I went for my first infusion at Stanford on Wednesday July 27th. Actually the procedure went really smoothly. I was there for about 6 hours; they always take the first infusion very slowly in case of any signs of side effects. After I was driven home feeling quite normal. In the meantime I had a second set of blood work done about a week before the infusion. The results were slightly better. The ANCA was of course still positive and the PR3 was 546, down from the previous reading of 750 but still very high. The CRP was back in the normal range but the kidney function tests were still abnormal as was the hemoglobin and hematocrit. My doctor interpreted this an indication that the high doses of steroids I had been given were working to reduce the inflammation.

The following week on August 5th I went back to Stanford for my second infusion but I never got it. The nurses typically monitor blood pressure and heart rate prior to giving the infusion and apparently my blood pressure was 170/90 and my heart was racing at around 120 to 130 beats per min. My normal resting heart rate was previously around 50 to 60 beats per min, which is low, because I swim laps daily. These problems with my heart really freaked out the medical staff and they admitted me into the cardiac unit. My doctor came to visit me and I told her about the other symptoms that I was experiencing. I seemed to be getting a fungal infection of my mouth which is quite common in patients undergoing treatment with high dose steroids. The steroids suppress the immune system and opportunistic infections like the yeast infection in my mouth frequently occur. In addition I was developing sores on my lips and in my mouth, probably due to herpes infections, again as a result of being immuno-suppressed by the steroids. I also felt a numbness and tingling in my toes and fingers and was developing blood blisters there also. These symptoms were probably due to the GPA which can give rise to neurological damage that frequently involve the extremities. I spent the next three days in Stanford where I shared a room with a patient who was dying from renal cancer and I got to enjoy his family coming in and discussing plans for his last days at home before his death! Really depressing and not what I needed in order to remain positive and deal with my own symptoms.

In the hospital room I had an iv in and was hooked up to a machine that measured my blood pressure and heart rate. At frequent intervals alarms connected to the equipment would go off and doctors and nurses would come in to check on me. The alarms indicated that my heart was racing and that I was producing numerous extra beats called pre-ventricular contractions or PVCs. Because of this I was given a beta blocker called metoprolol which is a drug that controls heart rate and slows it down. Every time the alarms would go off the nurses would come and ask me whether was I feeling ok and they seemed not to really believe me when I said I was! Actually what really concerned me were the constant alarms going off above my bed and the poor person I shared the room with who was groaning in agony during the night. It is perhaps no surprise that after three days of this I was really frazzled and the feeling of impending gloom and doom was almost too much to bear. It seems to me that the hospital staff, who otherwise did a really wonderful job, did not really understand the mental stress that I was experiencing during my stay. Sometimes this can be as bad as the condition that you are being treated for and I suspect it actually had a negative effect on me physically. During all the chaos incarnate that was swirling around me, I insisted that I be given my second Rituxan infusion and the doctors complied. So it was that I received the Rituxan late on my second day in the hospital with the doctor standing over me for the first 20 minutes looking extremely concerned. As usual we had the periodic alarm bells that went off but the procedure went pretty smoothly otherwise and I was relieved. After all of this I was released from Stanford on Saturday August 5th and was glad to be home.

My last set of blood tests in between all of this showed that there was still inflammation going on but more concerning to both my doctor and I was the fact that my creatinine levels were now way outside the normal range and creeping ever higher. This indicated that there was still kidney damage occurring and it did not bode well. Two weeks later my blood work showed that the creatinine levels were still rising and that my red blood cells and hematocrit still indicated that I was anemic but thankfully the PR3 levels had now come down to 109. For me the ANCA levels were always an indicator of my disease state so this data was at least good news as it indicated that the disease was responding to the Rituxan treatment. All of this however came at a price. The fungal infection in my mouth, the sores and blisters in my mouth and tongue, and the open wound on my upper lip made it extremely difficult if not impossible to eat. The high dose steroids were partly responsible for losing my sense of taste since I had already experienced this in my first bout with the disease. All of this was further exacerbated by the fungal infection in my mouth which, as I told my wife, made everything taste of shit! To treat the fungal infection I was put on an antifungal drug called ketoconazole (this did not really do anything so I was later given another anti-fungal called iconazole). The number of drugs I was taking was increasing daily and it is fair to say that they were all being used to treat various aspects of my symptoms, however, each drug that I was taking has side effects and it would be interesting at some point to speculate on the toll that all of this has on a body and organs that are already being ravaged by disease.

I existed on a diet almost exclusively of Haagen Daz Rich Chocolate ice cream shakes at 750 calories a shake. My goal was to try to at least maintain my weight, which had gone from 178 to 150 pounds during the course of my illness. The shakes at least were semi-palatable and I sucked them through a straw. Eating and chewing food was almost impossible because of the sores, every bite felt like I was eating razor blades. To try to get rid of the fungal infection I scraped my mouth and tongue several times a day, very painful, with a dilute solution of hydrogen peroxide. In addition my wife had collected a mouthwash from a compounding pharmacy that consisted of an antifungal agent, some lidocaine, which is used by doctors as a local anesthetic to numb the mouth, and a number of other agents. Similar mouthwashes are used by AIDS patients who are so immuno-compromised that they fall prey to similar and even worse mouth infections.

The only thing worse than all of this was the constant pounding of my heart and the tiredness and breathlessness of the atrial fibrillation. Before my illness I was a lap swimmer and would swim 50 laps non-stop in around 26 to 27 minutes almost daily. I also used to work out on a rowing machine and lift weights. Now I barely had enough energy to walk across the room and could maybe lift about 3 pounds in weights! In addition my muscle mass was wasting away thanks to my illness. During all of this I had my third and fourth Rituxan infusions at Sequioa Hospital in Redwood City. What a contrast to the Stanford experience. The nurses at Sequioa went about the infusion in a very calm and reassuring manner, even though at times my heart rate increased and my blood pressure went up slightly. All of this relaxed me and made me feel really comfortable. The subsequent infusions came and went and I went home without further incident each time.

Overcoming all of these horrors that were visited upon me required an absolutely iron will and a determined constitution. This I had in spades. I had overcome this disease once before and this time was going to be no different, I would beat it again. I made myself visualize mental images of my wife and children and family in the UK, including my parents and my sister who all were extremely worried about me. I had to survive for them also. When this was not enough I had photos of all of them on my iPhone and I would draw upon them for comfort and support. I would fight to survive and beat down the monster that was trying to destroy me. Instead I would destroy it. That became almost my daily mantra, I shouted out aloud to my reflection in the mirror of my bathroom - I WILL BLOODY BEAT THIS YOU #$%&*** EXPLETIVE DELETED. Good job nobody was watching this because they might have thought I was going insane!

Thus, it was that on August 31st I went back to Sequioa for my ablation surgery performed as before by Dr. Winkle who is a world expert in this procedure. He had warned me that the cure rate using this method was about 70% and this number reassured me. The surgery came and went and after an overnight stay at the hospital I went home. In the meantime the blood work that I had done two days previously was really positive. The kidney function tests were much better than before, although there was still protein in my urine indicating damage. I was told that eventually my kidney function could return to close to normal when the disease was in remission. Furthermore my ANCA titer was looking good and the PR3 reading was now only 107, down from an initial 751 at the height of the disease. Finally, my anemia was also getting better and the inflammation was also being well controlled reflected by the fact that my CRP readings were in the normal range again. Interestingly my blood sugar had gone up to levels that are pre-diabetic, a known side effect of the steroids that my doctor told me would disappear after I stopped taking the drugs. She was right, they did. Based on the fact that my disease was responding to the treatment, my doctor allowed me to start reducing the amount of steroids I was taking so that by early December I would be off them completely. I had already started reducing them and this had a beneficial effect on the fungal infection in my mouth which was starting to abate as were the sores in my mouth. The most stubborn sore, that on my lip, took almost a further month before it too was healed.

It looked like I was on the road to recovery and the only negative was that I was unable to fly over to the UK with my wife and son. My son who was doing a computer science and engineering degree at UC Santa Barbara had arranged to study abroad for one term and had elected to go to the University of Edinburgh. We had planned to go over as a family to visit my parents on the way and also to spend time with both my Brother-in-Law and his wife who were visiting London at this time, together with catching up with some good friends of ours who lived in Washington DC and were also in London for a few days. All of this was shot down in flames. I was so weak that I was in no position to fly out to the UK and so my wife would have to bear the strain and go over with my son. I in the meantime had to stay at home and miss out on a fabulous experience that I had been looking forward to for some time. To compound my misery even further, my Dad was not doing real well. He was in hospital with breathing problems brought on no doubt by his age: he was close to 90, and the many years that he had worked as a miner in the colliery. So my wife and son would get to visit him and I would not. The sheer frustration of all of this really had a negative mental affect on me but there was really nothing I could do but stay at home and work through my illness.

My mission for the remainder of September was to focus on getting well enough so that I could fly out to the UK in late November and spend time with my family and son. The plan was that I would take my son to a soccer match to see my team Manchester United play, and I would also would take my grandson Steven, who had indicated he would like to see a game. I also planned to go hiking in Derbyshire and I had visualized climbing Kinder Scout in Edale up the Nab and Ringing Roger, a total hike of 5 miles and an ascent of 1500 feet. An ambitious plan since at the present time all I could manage to climb were 3 steps in the house with an ascent of a few feet! But it was good to have a goal to aim at I needed this to continue for both my mental and physical recovery.

Thus it was that I spent the next 11 weeks doing exercises such as stair stepping, squats and lifting weights at least three times a week. I had lost so much muscle mass on my thighs that if I tried to squat I did not have enough energy to get back up again. However, slowly but surely with a combination of good nutrition (I was eating well now) and daily exercises, including lap swimming, I was recovering my strength. This was accompanied by my labs which by mid October looked really good. My ANCA was negative as was my PR3, there was no inflammation, and the anemia was almost normal. My kidney function tests although still abnormal were the best they had been since the disease started. The only blot on all of this fabulous recovery was that my heart was not cooperating. My cardiovascular doctor had given me an iRhythm monitor. This is a device about the size of a credit card that is attached to two detachable and disposable electrodes. I put this device on my chest to scan my heart twice a day for ECG activity. The data the device had recorded was then transmitted over a phone line (much like a Fax signal) to a monitoring center and from there it was sent to my doctor. The bad news was that my heart was showing signs of atrial fibrillation again, clearly the initial procedure had not worked and my doctor suggested that perhaps another ablation might help. This was planned for November the 1st. I wanted to ensure ample recovery time because I was planning to fly to the UK on November 22nd and come hell or high water, nothing was going to prevent that.

The ablation procedure went well as usual and I went home after an overnight stay. The doctor told me to continue monitoring my ECG activity and that he hoped that the operation had taken care of it. We would know with time whether the ablation had worked or not and if it hadn't, then I had two options. I could go on anti-arrhythmia medicines such as sodium channel blockers to control it, but these drugs were not that effective and had some pretty undesirable side effects. The other option was to go through a procedure called synchronized electrical cardioversion in which an electric shock is administered at an optimal moment during the cardiac cycle. My labs that were done during my hospital stay for the ablation procedure were pretty good, my B cells were absent, and so the Rituxan had worked as advertised. My kidney function tests were still abnormal but closer to normal than they been since I got the disease and the ANCA tests were negative. Based on all of this I felt well enough and confident enough to embark on a trip to the UK to visit my parents and my son who was in Edinburgh and enjoying his stay over there. My visit to the UK was wonderful and I did all of the things I had set out to do including hiking in Derbyshire. It was tiring but I was able to pretty much do what I had been able to do before the illness had started. In addition I finally came off the steroids in early December and this felt really good.

In January my heart was going back to its irregular rhythms and it appeared that the ablation had not been successful and thus the doctor proposed that I have the synchronized electrical cardioversion procedure. In late January it was with some apprehension that I went back to Sequioa to have this minor procedure. My doctor had told me this procedure was pretty trivial, but all I could think of was what I had seen of it on TV in patients requiring resuscitation after a cardiac arrest. Typically in hospital TV dramas the words "code blue" come booming over the loudspeaker indicating a medical emergency. This is followed by staff rushing in to the affected patient who is lying on a gurney in the emergency room with an arrested heartbeat. The doctor quickly applies two paddles to the patient's chest and shouts out "clear" in a loud voice as a massive electric current, around 1000 volts, is applied, jerking the patient's body into the air and hopefully shocking the heart back into life! In reality my procedure was nothing like this. I lay there in a hospital bed sedated out of my mind and asked my wife when are they going to do the procedure, to which she replied with obvious amusement, they already did it! I guess real life pales in comparison to TV drama. Anyway the procedure worked and the atrial fibrillation appears to have gone, my heart is in normal sinus rhythm and except for a few extra beats here and there is pretty much normal again.

Over the next nine months I have had blood work done every four months and by the beginning of September 2012 my B cells were just starting to creep back. The plan was to keep me in remission by giving me two doses of Rituxan at two weekly intervals and I had those in October 2012. My last set of labs were pretty normal: no anemia, no red blood cells in my urine, negative ANCA, no inflammation. My kidney function tests were still slightly below normal and confirmed that the damage that had been done by the disease would probably never be totally repaired. But the injuries were not life-threatening and as long as I had no further damage and could stay disease free, would probably not affect the quality of my life too much. In the 4 years or so after my initial relapse from GPA my life has returned to pretty much what it was before the relapse, I swim regularly, travel within the US and to Europe, and socialize with friends and family. What a contrast to the pretty sorry state that I was when the disease last struck. All I initially had wanted to do was just to curl up into a ball and die; however, I have a really strong positive constitution and it was that and obviously the drugs that I took that got me through this rough patch in my life.

Chapter 9 The Future for GPA treatment

The future looks pretty bright now for patients with GPA compared to where it was around 40 years ago. The combination of cytoxan and high dose steroids, nasty as this is in terms of side effects, have kept many patients with severe disease alive. As we have seen there are an increasing number of alternative drugs to cytoxan to treat GPA patients. For example drugs that act by suppressing immune function, such as methotrexate, azathioprine, or mycophenolate mofetil can be used to treat mild forms of the disease and are not as toxic as cytoxan. Such drugs usually induce remission (the complete absence of all signs of the disease). In addition the introduction of Rituxan about 5 years ago is going to have a massive influence in treating the disease, sparing patients the horrors of treatment with cytoxan. Beyond these drugs there are a whole array of potential new approaches to treat the disease that are still in the early stages of pre-clinical and clinical drug development. Many of these drugs are quite specific and target only one component of the immune response rather than being broadly immunosuppressive like cytoxan. This will obviously be advantageous since it will lessen the chance that patients who take these drugs will fall prey to the opportunistic infections that are so common when they are treated with strong immunosuppressive drugs.

A striking example of the type of new approaches that pharmaceutical companies are taking to treat GPA is provided by the Bay Area company Chemocentryx, which has an inhibitor of the complement C5a receptor program that is currently in phase II clinical trials. The complement system is a series of proteins produced by the liver that helps antibodies and immune cells like neutrophils and macrophages to destroy infectious microbes. The complement protein C5a is part of this system and exerts its effects through a cell surface C5a receptor. It appears that C5a primes neutrophils so that they can respond to ANCA produced by B cells. This induces cellular damage to the endothelial cells that are part of the lining of small blood vessels producing the inflammation and vasculitis that is such a hallmark of the disease. A number of animal studies have shown that animals that have been made deficient in the expression of the C5a receptor are protected from these damaging effects of the complement system. Thus it was rationalized that small molecule inhibitors of the C5a receptor might be beneficial in treating GPA by blocking neutrophil priming. Whether or not the data from the animal studies are relevant to the human disease remains to be seen but it does nevertheless offer some hope for more specific side-effect sparing therapies.

A further example of a specific GPA-directed therapy that is still in the clinical pipeline is provided by the biologic Alemtuzumab (also known as Campath and Lemtrada). Alemtuzumab is a monoclonal antibody to a protein found on the surface of T lymphocytes known as CD52. The antibody acts on T cells much the same way as Rituxan acts on B cells, it kills them. This effect is long lasting and the T cells can take up to 24 months or longer to fully repopulate. As Campath, the drug is already approved to treat various T lymphocyte leukemia's. In addition, as Lemtrada, it has recently undergone successful FDA approval for the treatment of another autoimmune disease, multiple sclerosis.

Recall that although T cells are not directly involved in the pathophysiology of GPA they play a major role in aiding and abetting the B cells to produce the ANCA that play an important role in neutrophil activation and aggregation giving rise to the inflammation and cellular damage in GPA. Thus one can predict that treatment of GPA patients with

Alemtuzumab should be beneficial in treating the disease. Currently the drug is in phase II clinical trials in GPA patients. One slight caveat with this approach is that the drug is pretty immunosuppressive as can be imagined by wiping out the T cell population, and there have been some cases of it inducing other autoimmune diseases such as Graves disease. There is also a risk of Immune thrombocytopenic purpura which is a clinical syndrome in which there is a decrease in the number of platelets that can lead to excessive bleeding that can be life-threatening.

Another approach in the clinic that targets T cells is aimed at blocking their activation. Recall that we had discussed earlier that MHC proteins on antigen presenting cells (APC) are responsible for presenting bits of foreign antigen to T cells to activate them. However for this process to be complete the T cell needs a co-stimulatory signal provided by the interaction of a protein on its surface called CD28 with a membrane protein called B7 present on APC like activated B cells for example. If this occurs the T cell is activated. In contrast if B7 engages a protein on the T cell called CD152 instead of CD28 this inhibits T cell activation. Think of this process as an "on off" switch for T cell activation.

Abatacept is a protein in which the CD152 molecule (the "off switch") has been fused to an IgG chain and it thus inhibits T cell activation. In a small 20 patient phase II clinical study carried out at the Cleveland clinic abatacept was well tolerated and was associated with a high frequency of disease remission and prednisone discontinuation. Based on these positive results a larger 150 patient study started enrolling in 2014 to determine the safety and potential efficacy of abatacept in nonsevere GPA.

Although the new therapeutic approaches for the treatment of GPA offer considerable hope for patients, real progress will only come when we start to understand how this dreadful disease is initiated. There are a number of outstanding questions that will need to be answered before we can make headway in this area however. These include, but are not limited to, determining the role of ANCA in disease initiation. For example why is disease in some patients so tightly correlated to ANCA levels whereas in others it appears to be independent? What triggers are responsible for initiating disease - genetic, environmental, infectious, stress, etc? What is the interplay of these factors in triggering disease, is it the same in all individuals? Would inhibition of proteinase 3 ameliorate disease? Are all forms of the disease identical in their initiation or does GPA resemble other autoimmune diseases, for example multiple sclerosis, that exist in different sub-types, and does this explain why some patients who relapse do not respond well to previous treatments that were initially successful in inducing remission? Luckily there are a number of researchers and clinicians that are attempting to answer these and other questions. Ultimately this research will benefit patients with GPA by making available numerous new medications to treat this autoimmune disorder, each small increase in knowledge gained from the mechanism of action of the drugs that are used to treat the disease will ultimately benefit patients by aiding in the design of newer, more specific and less toxic drugs. Compared to where we stood 50 years ago when the disease was almost certainly a death sentence things are looking remarkably bright now for patients with GPA.

Chapter 10 Final Words

I would like to end my narrative on a personal note. Although my 20 plus years of battling GPA has exacted a great physical toll on my body, mentally it has left me a stronger person than I ever was before I got the disease. Let me explain. Having to overcome the physical horrors and ravages of the disease requires an absolute iron will and constitution to survive. It would be all to easy to just give up and let go. However, the desire to live and enjoy my life with my family and close friends was strong enough for me to be able to conquer this terrible disease despite all its devastating symptoms.

Living with GPA has enabled me to recognize what is truly important in my life. I have let go of things that I now regard as inconsequential to my life. For example like many people I used to stress about finances worrying about having enough money to provide a good life for my family. Since my illness I have pushed these worries to the back of my mind. Sure it is important to have money to pay the bills but there is no point in obsessing over it and having it become a major issue in your life. For what use is money as you are lying there in a hospital bed contemplating the potential end of your life. I would gladly have given up every penny that I own if I could have avoided ever getting GPA!

Ego is also not important to life. As a scientist of international renown in my own particular area of research I was always super thrilled to present my work at international conferences to an audience of my peers. In addition I am very highly published as a scientist, over 180 papers many of which are in prestigious journals. Before my illness I was fiercely proud of these accomplishments but now I have put them into some perspective. Scientific papers are important in advancing scientific knowledge but all too often they are also a means for self glorification. A line in an old Elvis Costello song that goes "yesterdays news is tomorrows fish and chip paper" just about sums that up. What use fame and glory as you are lying there in a hospital bed contemplating the potential end of your life. I would gladly have given up every paper that I had ever published if I could have avoided ever getting GPA!

I have learned that the most important thing in my life over every other aspect of my being is my family. Getting this horrible disease and surviving it has reaffirmed that knowledge in spades. I have also learned, as a consequence of my illness, to let go of negative thoughts related to past events that were distressing in my life. Since these things happened and I cannot change them anyway what use is obsessing over them. Instead of asking myself why me why was all of this pain and misery heaped upon me I have just let it go and I am reminded of a quote that goes "I cannot change yesterday, I can only make the most of today and look with hope toward tomorrow". That sums up exactly how I feel. I got this terrible disease, I overcame it twice and I look forward with anticipation to living a full and fruitful life with my family.

41386601R00044

Made in the USA
Lexington, KY
11 May 2015